Navigat. o

A Journey to HeartSpace Parenting

Naomi Rodriguez

ISBN: 9781731046468

CONTENTS

CHAPTER 1: INTRODUCTION

How many of you have a child that when you tell them to lower their voice or be quiet, they get louder? Perhaps, instead of following your directions, they yell at you instead because you didn't say please. The more you ask, the more they protest. Perhaps you're so stressed out you are finding gray hairs in places you didn't know they could grow.

Welcome to the school of hard knocks of parenting! As the mother of a child with behavioral issues, I know what it's like to have those moments when you think, "What happened to my life?"

I knew if I was going to help my child, I first had to help myself. Having a special needs child can be overwhelming and can have a huge impact on the whole family. Sometimes, parents also struggle with the same issues, and the numbers are increasing of parents being diagnosed at the same time as their child. Marriages of the parents of special needs children are eighty to ninety percent likely to end in divorce, versus fifty percent of marriages without special needs children. There are so many moving parts to ADHD and family dynamics, as well as a ton of resources for nutrition, behavioral therapy, occupational therapy, and many more ways of trying to help families cope with this. I'd like to focus on just one, parenting your special needs child from your heart space.

What is a "heart space" exactly? It's when you are in touch with your emotions, your child's emotions, and are filled with empathy and compassion for the struggle that your child is dealing with. HeartSpace, for me, was when my heart broke wide open for my child. I realized that my child was suffering. I could feel his pain instead of feeling anger for what he was doing. This was his way of letting me know the world was a tough place for him. Instead of pushing him away, I embraced him. I learned to parent from my heart.

I needed to show my child compassion, respect, manners, empathy, and how to interact with others in a way that was acceptable for society in order for him to be able to fit in. We are not all born knowing what to do and what society expects of us, and interacting socially is something that requires us to be emotionally savvy.

On my journey, what I am learning is that there is a framework to life, and I chose to build my life with things like honesty, trust, respect, compassion, empathy, loyalty, responsibility, and commitment.

I am going to tell you about the lessons I have learned from living with my beautiful son. I have learned how to go from feeling burdened to feeling blessed, and I want to tell you how I did it.

CHAPTER 2: WHAT EXACTLY IS ADHD?

ADHD is a chemical imbalance in the brain. According to the NIMH (National Institute of Mental Health), some areas of the brain grow slower than others, causing the child to be up to three years behind in brain development. These areas are emotions, learning, and the ability to regulate emotions. There may be problems in everyday life, socially, academically, and emotionally. Fifty to seventy percent of children with ADHD also have a learning disability.

Children with ADHD often struggle to express what is going on with them. No two children are alike. ADHD is complicated to diagnose and it can be difficult to find the right combination of treatments. Social and emotional maturity comes naturally for eighty to eighty-five percent of the population, but for children with ADHD, things like regulating their emotions, being able to acquire their social skills, read social cues, and understanding the conversation and subtext must be taught along with compassion and empathy. Parents are the biggest role models to their children. The way parents show up in the world will teach our children to show up too. Parents are the mirror of who their child will become!

Areas that people with ADHD often struggle with:

1. Emotional Regulation – Having the ability to respond appropriately in situations that are positive and negative.

2. Starting Tasks – Being able to start an activity like cleaning your room, even if you just do part now and part later.

3. Planning – The ability to plan your day correctly and be the most effective without wasting time.

4. Organization of Things – Everything has a place; being able to keep those things in those places in life, work, and socially.

5. Time Management – Getting to school on time, allowing enough time to brush teeth, get dressed, and have breakfast without being rushed.

6. Time Awareness – How long will it take? How much time has passed?

7. Finishing What You Started – Finishing the homework you started at school.

8. Inhibition – Being able to control impulses and the behaviors they create. Person reacts at the moment for instant gratification without thinking things through.

8. Cognition/Flexibility/Transition – Being made aware time is over, being able to think about what they have to do next and change gears smoothly without a meltdown.

9. Skillful Way with Words/Command of Language – Being able to answer a question with multiple answers or a problem with multiple solutions.

10. Working Memory – Sending them to get something and they come back without it.

CHAPTER 3: MY STORY

I was thirty-seven weeks pregnant having contractions. My doctor examined me and said my blood pressure is too high, so it was time to schedule a C-section. We waited for my husband, Wayne, to get to the hospital. It was 7:28 pm on Wednesday, October 25th when Jonathan was born. It was love at first sight; he had my exact face when I was born, a head full of dark brown hair, slant eyes, a cute button nose, and full lips. They laid him on my chest and that is when all my dreams and aspirations started forming of who he would become, all the things he would do, and what I would do to help him get there. I had a plan and it was perfect.

Jonathan was a challenge right from the beginning. He was a beautiful baby, but he seemed to cry all the time. As he continued through to toddlerhood, his behavior got worse. I fielded all kinds of ideas from well meaning friends and family, even those who suggested more spankings and more discipline. I tried every suggestion, hoping something would help my son behave like I wanted him to. I began to fear taking him in public because meltdowns were the status quo.

When Jonathan was about three years old, I decided to put him in a Montessori preschool. I was drawn to the peacefulness and the child-led idea behind that form of education. After a couple of months, however, the owner of the school called me. She told me that Jonathan would not sit long enough for the teacher to finish the lesson and that he had even spat in her face. They wanted to meet and talk about the situation. When I met with her, she said, "I don't know how to help you" and suggested parenting classes and promised their unwavering support. However, I was also told, "if you don't do something about your son's behavior, you are going to have to take him out of this school". Needless to say, I left that meeting overwhelmed and crying. How do you get kicked out of preschool?

One time, I recall taking a family trip to Disney. The day ended with Jonathan screaming so hard that when we left the park, security actually stopped us to check our ID's to make sure we weren't kidnapping him. We left, feeling humiliated and defeated.

I would lie in bed at night and wonder what kind of future he would have. I was so caught up in the anger and frustration of his behavior that I started to feel like he was ruining my life. Why do other parents get easy kids and I get a difficult one?

As time went on, I realized that we needed help navigating these waters. I used my medical background to help find providers who would support our journey. I also had to do some major work on MYSELF. What could I do as a parent that would help my child function in this world without so much strife? What could I do for myself and my marriage to help me deal with this stress? I knew there had to be a better way to deal with things than what we were doing, but my journey had just begun.

CHAPTER 4: WHY PARENTS WITH ADHD CHILDREN STRUGGLE TO FIND A LOVING, PEACEFUL PARENTING RELATIONSHIP WITH THEIR CHILDREN

Let's be real: having a child with ADHD can be one of the most frustrating things to a parent. Many things that come easily to most people were difficult for Jonathan, and by extension, made my life difficult. I often found myself feeling frustrated with him instead of seeing him for the child he was. He was struggling everyday and didn't know how to express it except to act it out in frustration -- the same frustration I was showing him. I had to learn how to calm down before I approached him. I learned to take a look at myself and the mirror I was holding up for my son. What did he see when he saw me angry and frustrated?

I began to realize that the anger and frustration actually came from my hurt and disappointment of not having the child I expected. I had to mourn the unrealistic dream of who I thought he should be. I needed to accept who he was and work with the child that was screaming that his world was too hard for him. I began to approach my child with an open heart and compassion for his difficulties and an understanding that he was doing the best he could. I saw that he needed me to meet him where he was, not where I expected him to be. It was time to stop trying to fit a square peg into a round hole; it just wasn't going to fit.

I also realized that I was withholding my physical love from my child due to my own frustration. It was hard for me to love him through his tantrums and frustration. I realized that the behavior was not who he was, it was something he did when he didn't know what else to do. I began to see that what I was doing and how I was behaving was affecting my child. Once I started to break it all down and remove the frustration from my parenting, I was able to understand and have compassion for my child and his struggles.

He was feeling out of control inside, and he needed to feel a sense of security. What I see with my son is that he needs for me to sit with him and hug him and kiss him every single day. It helps him to feel the love that I have for him, even through the toughest times.

CHAPTER 5: KEY SKILLS FOR PARENTS

Defiant behavior is a symptom of an underlying problem. Regulating emotions goes hand in hand with behavior. My experience has been that first comes the thought, then comes the feeling, and then the reaction.

Here are some key skills you can focus on to help keep yourself calm and reach your child at the heart level:

Emotional Regulation & Self Care - Checking in with yourself. How am I feeling today? What have I done for myself today?

Perspective Taking - Is this a big deal? A battle worth fighting?

Find the teachable moments when things are quiet and create bonding time with your child. It's hard to reach someone when they are frustrated and upset. Wait for the quiet moments to address things and help them understand what went wrong, what went right, and what can be improved upon.

Offer some power and autonomy by letting your child have a voice to be heard and understood. Give them choices and respect their decisions.

Clean up the mess when you lose your cool. Offer genuine apologies and explain to your child the ways you could have reacted differently to the situation.

Life is about being good at problem solving. When decisions are made, they have to be made from a rational state of mind, not an emotional state of mind. Our emotional regulation (i.e: our ability to self soothe) holds all of our power. If we are frustrated, stressed, tired, hungry, or overwhelmed then we create more distance. Emotions are contagious, thus we want to ensure that we are not adding to the stress due to our verbal and nonverbal cues. Be mindful of your words, actions, and temperament in front of your child. Save your meltdowns and venting for a trusted friend or care provider or for when you are alone. It's normal to get frustrated and even angry, but try your best to maintain emotional balance in front of your child as much as possible. Be the model for them!

Here's an acronym I made up (using my nephew's name) to help me remember how to deal with kids during the toughest of times:

E- Embrace the child and situation.
V- Validate feelings; they are real and powerful.
O- Observe the child and your own struggles and get professional help.
N- Never forget their struggles are a cry for help.

CHAPTER 6: CHALLENGE TO PARENTS

My hope is to empower parents with special needs children.

I challenge them to ask themselves -- what are the lessons our children are here to teach us?

In the midst of my darkest times, when no one could help me, I would pray at night for God to reveal the lessons that my son was here to teach me. After months of praying, the answer came in the form of a 30 minute tantrum. What I saw in the eyes of my child was that he was suffering. In that suffering, I saw a child that was screaming for help. I realized that what he was here to teach me were lessons of compassion, empathy, kindness, and how to love unconditionally without judgment.

I spent my time attending support groups and talking to parents online and in person. I also spent hours doing one-on-one sessions with a Parenting Coach that helped me understand that if I allowed my emotions to control my reactions, I was coming from a place of anger and frustration instead of a place of understanding and unconditional love for what my child was going through. I had to change what I was doing and approach him with an open heart from a place of love. Once I understood that, when a problem occurred, I had to take note of how I was feeling. Was I having a bad day? Was I empty with no more to give? The parenting coach taught me how important self care is, in showing up to be present for my child. My thought was, ok, now how do I find the time for self care? In my busy days of working and taking him from one appointment to another, I didn't know where to start. She suggested starting with five minutes a day for a week. I have a book called "Illuminata: A Return to Prayer" by Marianne Williamson, and I knew I could do that in five minutes. As I spent time reading prayers over a period of time, my heart started to soften for my child. I started to see him through a different lens. He was struggling, and he needed my help. He wasn't being "bad" or acting out on purpose. He needed guidance and support, and as his parent, it was up to me to give him those things.

Things to remember when your child is acting out:

- This is not a reflection of you or your parenting, this is a child asking for help
- Ground yourself, feel your feet on the floor. If you are feeling grounded and calm, your child will see you as a safe person, even as they are coming apart
- Take a TIME OUT for yourself. Spend 5-10 minutes breathing and checking in with yourself before interacting with your upset child. Be the voice of reason and calm for them. They are counting on you to help them.
- Find something you can do for 5 minutes a day that is JUST FOR YOU. What brings you joy? What gives you peace? What inspires you? Chase these things!

CHAPTER 7: 7 STEPS TO MANAGING YOUR ADHD CHILD

Unfortunately, there is not one easy solution to help every child, but I've found these steps to be useful in helping both my son with his diagnosis as well as helping me as a parent with how to help him:

1. Recognize - One of the first steps is UNDERSTANDING YOUR CHILD'S PATTERNS. On the outside, my son's behavior seemed random and disjointed, but once I started paying attention, I started to notice a pattern. For example, when recess is over and it's time to go back to class, he will start yelling that he's not ready to leave yet. Like a detective looking for clues, a pattern began to emerge. My son had problems transitioning, going from one thing to another. I came up with a plan to help him when it was time to transition to something new. I would tell him where we were going and explain to him how much longer we would be there. After doing it for a little bit, he started to get it.

By UNDERSTANDING THE PATTERN, I then could anticipate his behavior and hopefully be a couple of steps ahead of him. This gave me the opportunity to stop being a reactive screaming machine and think before I reacted. Instead of seeing him as an out-of-control child, I started to see him as a child who could not control his emotions, and I was able to find empathy for him.

I stopped being angry with him for his behavior. I started to ask myself how he must be feeling. He must feel so out of control. Now when I see the behavior changing, I engage him by talking to him about how he is feeling.

Watch your child and see if you can understand their pattern. It doesn't work to force them to fit into your idea of what they should be. What works is UNDERSTANDING your child's world - so, watch, listen, and love them.

2. Ask for Help from Professionals & Other Parents - Seek out support groups and playgroups with others with ADHD. Join online communities and groups that deal with ADHD. Both you and your child will feel less alone once you find a good support network.

3. Get to Know Your Resources - Talk to your insurance provider and seek out free/inexpensive options in your area. Investigate your care providers and seek out alternative treatment options as well (nutrition, holistic care options, acupuncture, occupational therapy, traditional therapy, eastern medicine). Yes, there are a lot of snake oil salesmen out there, and yes, it can be a crazy journey, but this is where you'll find the most value from your network. Find out what has been working for others and see if its an option/good fit for your family.

4. Create a Plan and Commit To It - (see the next section on creating a plan)

5. Practice Gratitude - This is a great habit to get into as a family. During family time, dinner time, car rides, or even as a part of nightly journaling, each family member should make a list of things they are grateful for. This seems like a small thing, but it can really offset the frustration and anger that can boil up and reminds us to focus on what's really important.

6. Practice Self Care & Self Awareness - What can you do, as parents, to support yourself and each other? This may be carving out time for exercise or fun activities/hobbies, spending time with friends, seeking therapy/counseling, or eating better. There are lots of ways to take care of oneself, but we've all heard the warning to put oxygen masks on ourselves before our kids. We need to help ourselves first, so that we can be the support pillars that our children need. Knowing when you are about to reach your breaking point is an important part of this work. What can you do to calm yourself? What works for you to move into a forward-thinking mindset rather than focusing on the problem? What things do you enjoy? What things help you feel more centered? Group and individual therapy, other parents, and online groups are great resources to learn these things about yourself. Make the time for it, you won't regret it!

7. Work As A Team (Family/Community) - Bring everyone in your child's life into the fold. Explain to them what patterns you've noticed, what seems to work, what seems to make things worse, what everyone's role is, and how everyone can work together to help this child thrive. For example, if your child's nutritionist suggests a certain diet, make sure that he's not going to Grandma's and filling up on cupcakes. If the therapist suggests sensory toys, then bring your child's teacher into that conversation and see if they can be on board. YOU are your child's biggest advocate and while it can be challenging to coordinate your team efforts, it really will go a long way in helping your child have a stable and supportive environment.

CHAPTER 8: HOW TO CREATE A PLAN WITH YOUR CHILD

Getting your child to be an active participant in his or her own life is a huge step towards problem-solving and independence. Oftentimes, when I've hit a wall on how to help my son deal with challenges, I sit down and create a plan with him.

Step 1: Share with your child the need to figure out a way this works for everyone. Ask them if we can negotiate a resolution.

Step 2: Capture the details of your agreement. Come up with options and guidelines for the situation at hand. How would they like to handle it? How much flexibility do they need or are you willing to offer? What are the consequences of breaking the agreement? Role play the options with your child and listen to their input and suggestions and incorporate them into the plan.

Step 3: Set your kids up for success! Ensure you have consistent, eye-level discussions and use simple reminders without lecturing. Visual aids and charts can be helpful here too!

Step 4: Deal with your own emotions when you feel guilty and remind yourself of why you created this agreement. It's easy to give in when you are feeling frustrated or desperate. Hang onto your serenity and your plan!

Step 5: Get down to kids' eye level, ask if they remember the agreement which is printed on the wall. Watch your nonverbal cues as well. Remind them that they helped create it and point out what the next steps will be.

Step 6: Try to put yourself in your child's shoes. Tell them a story/anecdote from your own life to show that you understand their pain and frustration and explain how you dealt with it. If you didn't deal with it well, share that and what you would've done differently. The goal here is to show and feel empathy for your child and to gain trust as a foundation in your relationship.

CHAPTER 9: MISTAKES TO AVOID

What I've come to realize is that ADHD is a mental disorder as well as a learning disability. If I tell people that my son has dyslexia, which is a learning disability, I seem to receive compassion, but if I say he has ADHD, I tend to feel judged about my parenting. What some people don't understand is the complexity of ADHD/ADD and the fact that 50% to 70% of children with the disorder have a learning disability and struggle with emotional regulation. We see children in school struggling with behavioral issues and the root of the problem ends up being a learning disability or a sensory disorder. What we see is a result of their frustration from their inability to learn at the rate of everyone else or in the same environment as everyone else. With one in five being diagnosed, chances are there could be four to six children struggling in one class with one teacher.

I want to share what my friend, mentor, and parent coach, Rhea Lalla wrote and gave me permission to share with all of you:

"When you create trust and intimacy consistently with your child, you become a parent who can calm your kids down, get your kids to listen, and encourage your kids to share everything about their life openly and often, without boundaries. When this occurs, you have the privilege to witness the intricacies of their fears, passions, hurts, and hopes and intuitively you'll both know something magical is occurring.

So before I tell you the secret to creating this kind of openness, I need you to imagine the most heartbreaking, stressful situation you've had with your child.

Here's some examples of what children say....

- I hate myself
- I hate you
- I hate my brother/sister
- I don't like school
- I'm not good at that/anything
- You like (insert sibling) more than me

Perhaps it's something they did, such as....

- Hit people or you
- Break things in the home
- Continuously do things that annoy you
- Throw things
- Tantrum in public
- Storm upstairs screaming

When these things happen, you may feel panic, desperation, anger, or even sadness. You immediately want to fix, defend, argue, question, and you can sense tension, anger, frustration, sadness in your body. So do your kids!

Now....what you do next will determine every future interaction you have with your child. In that crucial moment, you have the power to close the conversation down with your response. You might unwittingly restrict their openness and future honesty with guilt, shame, or blame. However, there is a better way...

I'd like you to try a new move.

No matter what your child says, believe in your heart and mind it's 100% justified and reasonable. They may say or do the most outrageous, horrible, frightening or hurtful thing. Still, trust there is some kernel of truth and validity to what they said, felt and did.

This means if your child says something extreme like "I hate you"...

Do not say:

- That hurts me (which creates guilt in your child and shuts conversations down)
- Well, I'm sorry you feel this way (which shows indifference and no desire to understand their pain)
- It's not nice to hate (which is judgmental and shames your child)
- You wouldn't like it if someone said that to you (doesn't change a future behavior, makes your child feel guilty)
- That's a mean thing to say (which shames them and confirms you don't understand them)
- Why would you say such a thing? (again, guilt and won't solve any of the difficult feelings they are experiencing)
- How about a time out!? (threatens, this dismisses the situation and punishes without trying to understand your child)
- You haven't seen anything yet! (threatens and shows vindictiveness)
- Some other defensive, angry rant which adds fuel to the fire, aggravates your child, and leaves you feeling angry, resentful, and later on, guilty.

Instead try this:

(Energetically, make the switch and go into a loving and curious detective mode)

- I'm really interested in learning about what happened here, please tell me more.
- I can imagine you're in a great deal of pain right now, and I must have done something to upset you. I want to see how I can fix it.
- I can imagine you must be very angry right now. I know when I've felt like someone wasn't listening to me, I didn't like them too much either.
- Sometimes I do and say things that aren't the best. Mommy/Daddy are learning new moves all the time. Can you teach me how I can love you better?

When you do this, your kids feel understood on their level. They also feel safe, which brings their defenses down. They'll then open themselves up and become trusting. But to do this well, we must hold all the attributes of a good detective. We must have a deep desire to transcend whatever conscious or unconscious thoughts, biases, and blind spots we have that keep us reactive instead of responsive.

The beauty is, if we can do this (and we can!), we'll raise the maturity of ourselves along with our kids. Through these interactions, we'll uncover our own emotional issues and unhealthy thought patterns and begin to heal our own wounds from our childhood that haunts our behavior as parents.

Ultimately, we can use these opportunities to become our highest selves, so our kids can do the same."

Rhea Lalla - Founder, buildgreatminds.com

CHAPTER 10: RESOURCE LIST

(I used the lessons I learned in these courses to write this book)

My website for HeartSpace Parenting: http://www.togetherforallofus.com

For those that live in Los Angeles, UCLA has some of the best programs in the nation that address children and young adults that suffer with mental and behavioral health issues.

www.semel.ucla.edu/peers www.uclahealth.org/ABCChild

www.semel.ucla.edu/adc/ocd www.semel.ucla.edu/socialskills

www.semel.ucla.edu/autism/clinic

UCLA Executive Function Educational Training UCLA-parenting-Childrens-Friendship-Program.pdf

National Institute of Mental Health https://www.nimh.nih.gov/index.shtml

National Resources on ADHD for Adults and Children https://chadd.org

Learning Disabilities Association of America https://ldaamerica.org/types-of-learning-disabilities/

Additude Magazine https://www.additudemag.com/

CHAPTER 11: FINAL THOUGHTS

My journey hasn't been an easy one, and I know that there will be many more days of fighting an uphill battle. What I have today that I didn't have before is HOPE. I would like to share the HOPE I have found with YOU as you move through your own journey. Learning how to regulate my own emotions and how to show my child unconditional compassion, empathy, and respect has been a huge learning curve, but one with which I am starting to finally get comfortable. Going from feeling burdened to feeling blessed has changed my entire perception of myself, my child, and the world as a whole. I find myself having more compassion for other parents and children as they move through their own struggles, whether I know what they are or not. My hope for you is that you move forward with your children and yourselves, do the work, dig deep, and reclaim the love and joy that was meant for your family.

If you are interested in one-on-one coaching or having me speak at your event, please contact me here:

http://www.togetherforallofus.com/
https://www.facebook.com/togetherforallofus

ACKNOWLEDGEMENTS

This book has been the birth of my HeartSpace, the space from which my son was born. He has became my greatest teacher of unconditional love and I will love you always. To Evon Rodriguez, you were my first baby and I will always love you like my son. To my parents, Percy & Jose (Joe) Rodriguez, for providing Jay and I a safe place to grow and loving us unconditionally without judgement. To my brother, Jay Rodriguez, I love you more than you know! To my husband, thank you for your support, I love you very much! To Lora Denton, thank you, thank you for taking all my words and giving them life. Having undiagnosed ADHD and dyslexia this has been an amazing journey for me. I remember that in school ,I could not write an essay and now here is my first book! Rhea Lalla, thank you for showing me how to be present in my parenting and how parents choose the relationship they have with their children. And last but not least, I want to thank Judy Carter, Author, Speaker, Teacher, and a very funny lady with a beautiful heart that guided me on how to take my mess and make it my message.

Love, Peace, & Great Health to all!

Love,

Naomi

ABOUT THE AUTHOR

Naomi Rodriguez – Parent, Mentor, Advocate

I am a proud mother of a thirteen year old boy who struggles with ADHD. He has taught me that his struggles are real and that ADHD is real. My son has been my greatest teacher of Love, Empathy, Compassion, and Kindness. When the parent becomes the student, the child becomes the teacher!

I am the recipient of The President Volunteer Service Award presented by the President's Council on Service and Civic Participation in recognition and appreciation of commitment to strengthening our nation and making a difference through volunteer service at Burbank Boulevard Elementary 2011.

I've also participated in the following programs:

2010 CHADD Certificate of Achievement Parent to Parent:
  Family Training on ADHD
2011 UCLA Parent Training Friendship Program
2013 UCLA Parent Training ABC Program
2016 Graduate of the Special Needs Network Parent Advocacy
  Mentor Program
2017 UCLA Program on Executive Function
2018 Build Great Minds Academy Certificate of Completion of
  The Parent Coaching Program

Made in the USA
Middletown, DE
25 May 2023

31475654R00019